~It is not easy

To apologize

To begin over

To admit error

To take advice

To be unselfish

To be charitable

To be considerate

To keep on trying

To avoid mistakes

To forgive and forget

To keep out of the rut

To make the most of a little

To maintain a high standard

To recognize the silver lining

But it always pays

Charlotte Albina Aikens

CHARLOTTE'S RULES

FOR

NURSES

A Centennial Celebration

Charlotte Aikens
adapted by Lois Angelo

LCCN: 9780692418987

ISBN: 1511694564.
ISBN-13: 978-1511694568

Preface

How the world has changed in the 100 years since Charlotte Aikens wrote her classic textbook, "Studies in Ethics for Nurses." Televisions did not exist, movies did not talk, there were few telephones and radios, Model T cars were starting to roll off assembly lines, women were not allowed to vote, and World War I was raging in Europe.

With the rapid immigrant migration from Europe, major cities were impoverished with huge amounts of inadequate tenement housing. Housing shortages, sanitation issues, significant mortality caused distress for many. Healthcare for most of the population was inadequate. (Judd 2010) The major causes of death were heart disease, tuberculosis, pneumonia, and acute nephritis-Bright's disease. (US Department of Commerce, 1918)

The vast majority of nursing students, white and female, set out to earn a diploma while living and "training" in a hospital. They were considered "probationers" during their first year of study. The nurse was subjected to periods of long and exhausting mental strain along with much hard physical work. "Modern Hospital" deplored the presence of disreputeable hospitals in a ringing 1914 editorial: "Many hospitals are a disgrace to everybody connected with them. Some are notorious abortion "parlors," some are distinguished by a reputation for shady transactions in their financial dealings." The October 1913 issue of Ladies' Home Journal published a scathing criticism of the manner in which hospitals fed their student nurses in 7 out of 10 hospitals. All across the nation there was concern over the decreasing numbers of nurse-training applications and the slipping personal standards of those who did apply. Between 1908 and 1917, there was a surge of protective legislation when 39 states passed new laws or strengthened old ones regulating the hours of women's work. (Kalisch 1995)

Now, 100 years later, with massive scientific and technological advances in all aspects of American life, including the ongoing transformation of healthcare, "Studies in Ethics for Nurses", remains vital, continuing to breathe life into the core values and behaviors for nursing today. It reflects virtue ethics, which date back to the writings of Plato and Aristotle and is the concern for the moral, personal well-being and actions of the nurse. It was the dominant methodology of nursing ethics from the 1800s to the late 1950s, lost some influence after the early 1960s with the domination of other philosophical frame-works within the burgeoning field of bioethics, but lately it is recovering ground in nursing ethics. (Hellyer 2007) Virtue ethics with its focus on a person's character, can provide a holistic analysis of moral dilemmas in nursing and facilitate flexible and creative solutions. (Arries 2005) Also, virtue ethics can be used as a framework for nurse educators to teach nursing students how to contribute to the development of healthy workplaces by engaging in respectful relationships with their clients and colleagues. (Russell 2014)

"Charlotte's Rules for Nurses", a concise, reorganized version of "Studies in Ethics for Nurses", retains basic nursing concepts and the strong emphasis on how virtue ethics affect patient care. Contemporary, dynamic issues are included, such as patient confidentiality, professional boundaries, anger in nursing, mind-body relationships, nurses' health, bullying, personal finances and even touches on what is now known as cognitive behavioral treatment. As men in nursing were extremely rare, the nurse is always referred to as "she." Chapters, pages and paragraphs have been deleted from the original textbook, particularly those relating to the details of training schools, hospital economy, and private duty home care. However, no additional words have been added. Every word belongs to Charlotte Aikens.

Charlotte Albina "Lottie" Aikens (1868-1949) born in Canada and a graduate of Ontario's Stratford Hospital was a widely known nursing authority. An Army nurse in the Spanish-American War, Miss Aikens was an educator, supervisor of nurses, an active member of the American Hospital Association, and as the director of Sibley Memorial Hospital in Washington, DC, advocated for a strong theoretical foundation in the nurses' training school. She wrote several textbooks on nursing, nursing education and hospital administration and helped set up Detroit's home nursing program.

Nurses at every level of education will enjoy and benefit

from Aikens' wisdom and passion for nursing in "Charlotte's Rules for Nurses." It can enhance introductory courses, later applied to clinical experiences in various specialty and leadership courses, and continue as a resource for personal growth in nursing. Instructor materials, including a slide presentation and a test bank of multiple choice questions, are available on request.

Here's to Charlotte Aikens and the hope that her vision for nursing will live on for at least another 100 years!

Arries, E (2005) Virtue Ethics: An Approach to Moral Dilemmas in Nursing. *Curationis* 28 (3), 64-72.

Hellyer, J (2007) *The Good Nurse*. Doctoral Dissertation, University of Iowa, Religious Studies, 4-5.

Judd, D et al (2010) *A History of American Nursing*, Boston: Jones and Bartlett, 64.

Kalisch, P & Kalisch B (1995) *The Advance of American Nursing*. 3rd edition, Philadelphia: Lippincott, Williams, Wilkins, 205- 210.

Russell, MJ (2014) Teaching Civility to Undergraduate Nursing Students using a Virtue Ethics-Based Curriculum, *Journal of Nursing Education*, 53 (6) 313-319.

Treasure, E (1943) *The Origin, Growth and Development of the Lucy Webb Hayes National Training School Including Sibley Memorial Hospital*, MSN Dissertation, Catholic University of America, 16, 32.

US Department of Commerce (1918), *Mortality Statistics 1916*, 17th annual report, 21

Lois Angelo, APRN

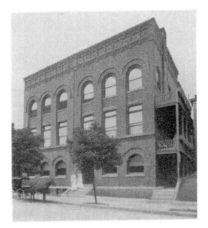

Sibley Memorial Hospital in Washington, DC, circa 1900, when Charlotte Aikens was director of the hospital and the training school. After the workload became too heavy for the nursing students to attend all of the theoretical classes, Miss Aikens adopted a curriculum for the preparation of "professional nurses." Her administration was very efficient, and the hospital became well known for the excellent service to its patients. (Treasure 1943) Photo courtesy of Robert Sloan, Sibley Hospital.

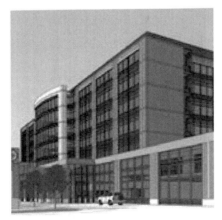

Sketch of the new Sibley Memorial Hospital to be completed in 2016. Photo courtesy of Robert Sloan.

FOREWORD

The purpose of this textbook is to emphasize the importance of ethical training and *to make nurses think*, think hard and frequently about questions of conduct and duty as it relates to nursing life. The ideals of character and service which a nurse holds will greatly influence her practical work every day of her nursing career.

The entrance of the nurse candidate into the new world of the hospital is a rather bewildering experience, and the process of adjusting herself to these new conditions, laws, and customs is rarely easy. It is easy in the pressure of training school to devote all one's time to the technical part of a nurse's training and allow ethical training to be crowded out. Yet no amount of devotion to the technical instruction will ever compensate for failure to give the nurse proper rules and principles of guidance in the moral realm; no amount of other classes will make up to a nurse what she loses, if the culture of character is forgotten during her training. Conditions making it impossible for the careful selection of candidates that was possible in the earlier years of training schools, call for more systematic and careful ethical teaching than has been customary.

What is most needed is that the student should meditate on the ethical questions likely to confront a nurse, and the lessons applied to her own experiences. It is the author's conviction that ten minutes of serious reflection on ethical principles involving concrete problems will accomplish more in impressing them with the importance of right decisions than hours of lectures on abstract virtues–lectures in which the nurse is simply a passive agent, expected to absorb instruction. Lectures cannot too soon be abandoned in the teaching of ethics, if worthwhile results are to be expected. The requiring of written personal opinions to decide ethical questions is a valuable method in the teaching of ethics. Nurses should be trained to think things through to a logical conclusion and to be able to give reasons why they reached decisions.

The practical problems used in the book are drawn from life, and each teacher can add to them or substitute from her own experience. The author makes no apology for revealing certain ethical failures, believing that only by the frank recognition of existing weaknesses can the weak points be strengthened; only by bringing the results of ethical failures into an open forum for discussion can conditions be improved. The only way common ethical failures can ever be corrected is by instilling in the heart of every nurse a desire to be true to her own best self; by giving each individual nurse higher standards of life and conduct, and showing her how she may reach those standards.

If this book helps in any measure toward bringing the ethical training and practice of nurses nearer to the ideals of life and conduct which Florence Nightingale has given to the world, it will have accomplished its mission.

During the preparation of this volume, the textbooks, Principles of Ethics by Bowne, Social Law of Service by Ely, have been studied. Other books referred to have been, Constructive Ethics by Courtney, Outlines of Ethics by Dewey, The Ethics of Personal Life by Griggs, and Nursing Ethics by Robb.

Charlotte A. Aikens
Detroit, Michigan
1916

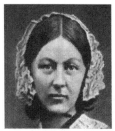

Florence Nightingale, about 1858
Born in Florence, Italy, May 12, 1820. Died in London, England, August 13, 1910.

~~~~~~

SANTA FILOMENA
By Henry Wadsworth Longfellow
In honor of Florence Nightingale

Whene'er a noble deed is wrought,
Whene'er is spoken a noble thought,
  Our hearts, in glad surprise,
  To higher levels rise.

The tidal wave of deeper souls
Into our inmost being rolls,
  And lifts us unawares
  Out of all meaner cares.

Honor to those whose words or deeds
Thus help us in our daily needs,
  And by their overflow
  Raise us from what is low!

Thus thought I, as by night I read
Of the great army of the dead,
  The trenches cold and damp,
  The starved and frozen camp,

The wounded from the battle-plain,
In dreary hospitals of pain,
  the cheerless corridors,
  The cold and stony floors.

Lo! in that house of misery
A lady with a lamp* I see
  Pass through the glimmering gloom,
  And flit from room to room.

And slow, as in a dream of bliss,
The speechless sufferer turns to kiss
  Her shadow, as it falls
  Upon the darkening walls.

As if a door in heaven should be
Opened, and then closed suddenly,
  The vision came and went,
  The light shone was spent.

On England's annals, through the long
Hereafter of her speech and song,
  That light its rays shall cast
  From portals of the past.

A lady with a lamp shall stand
In the great history of the land,
  A noble type of good,
  Heroic womanhood.

Nor even shall be wanting here
The palm, the lily, and the spear,
  The symbols that of yore
  Saint Filomena** bore.

~~~~~~

The Atlantic Monthly; November 1857; *"Santa Filomena,"* by Henry Wadsworth Longfellow ; Volume 1, No. 1; pages 22-23.
* first use of phrase " A lady with a lamp" in reference to Florence Nightingale.
**St. Filomena is a Catholic patron of health/illness.

Contents

1 Ethics 1

2 Hospital Atmosphere 7

3 Loyalty 11

4 Everyday Routine 15

5 Honesty 21

6 Carelessness 25

7 Conversation 29

8 Tact 33

9 Imagination 37

10 Judgment 41

11 The Nurse Herself 47

12 Types of Nurses 63

13 The Nurse's Health 69

14 Developing a Symmetrical Life 79

15 After Graduation 85

16 The Head Nurse 93

17 A Nurse and Her Money 99

18 The Pioneer Spirit 103

1

ETHICS

Ideals and standards must change and grow as civilization advances and knowledge is increased, but the foundation principles do not change. These are based on the world-old law of good will, of love of one's neighbor, of the duty to promote the general welfare of all concerned. The subject of ethics enters into the secret places of one's life. Ethics does not concern itself simply with ideals and virtues. The subject is as broad and deep as life itself. Dictionaries define ethics as the science which deals with moral conduct or with human duty.

As related to nursing, ethics has to do with the ideals, customs and habits accumulating around the character of the nurse. The ethics of personal life affect the very center of all efforts for the improvement of nurses and nursing, what she does and is, and the influence she is exerting affects the whole nursing structure. Ethical questions are practical questions. They are questions dealing with the conduct of each nurse, with her way of looking at situations and of dealing with them as they present themselves in a more or less monotonous tone day after day.

The sense of duty is much stronger in some individuals than in others. One person sees a duty of common humanity and is impelled to perform it. Another sees the same thing, but has no feeling that he has any moral obligation to concern himself in any way about it. To make a reputation for being faithful and dependable is possible for every nurse and means still more in the years to come. In a long career, the nurse's ideals of conduct and of duty are the biggest factors in her success, professionally and financially.

INTEGRITY

Integrity is that spirit of whole-hearted honesty, which excludes all forms of injustice that might favor one's self. It has special reference in matters which cannot well be reached by laws or rules that a nurse's self of honor will be tested, in carrying out obligations in the right way, even though no one but the nurse herself may ever know of the matter which involved the question of honor. To be true to one self, to one's own best ideals, is the hardest task a nurse will ever undertake.

Carrying out the letter of the law or rule, but deliberately violating the spirit of it, is a temptation which comes to every nurse at some time. It is one which involves the nurse's personal sense of honor. To do a thing or to refrain from doing it, simply because one is trusted, is a real test of character.

Reliability

The work of the world depends upon reliable people and this is especially true of hospital work, where life and death issues often hinge upon some apparently small thing. Being reliable is not easy surface work. It takes day after day, year after year of picking up the threads that the careless drop, of being ready in emergencies where others fail, of doing uninteresting work that others tire of. It takes all this to make the dependable man and woman known and valued.

Will

The nurse's will, the power of the mind by which she decides to do or not to do, is the great test of character and life. The training of the will until right habits are formed, and certain courses are taken, or things done unconsciously or without effort of will is at the bottom of character building. Results are shown in what a nurse does, not what she thinks or intends. We are influenced, partly unconsciously, to the formation of habits by the example and influence of those with whom we live in daily contact and especially by the example of those in authority. Our attitude of mind is influenced by their attitude, but our wills are given to us to help keep us from forming wrong habits of body or of mind. We may love people without copying their faults.

RESPONSIBILITY

In the hospital, individuals are valued largely according to their ability to carry responsibility. The ease and effectiveness with which a nurse is able to assume responsibility determines her value in large measure. This fact cannot be too strongly emphasized. The nurse who feels personal responsibility is the nurse who is trusted and depended on, and who, later, has larger responsibilities committed to her.

A system of semi-military discipline prevails in the hospital. The nurse is expected to observe the orders and rules given to those to whom authority has been delegated, whatever her personal feelings toward the individual may be. Each worker is expected to be in his own place until relieved from duty; to attend to the responsibilities assigned to him and who will do the things ordered at the proper time, and if they find it impossible to carry out an order, they will, at once, report it to those in authority.

Most of the rules and customs in hospitals are designed directly or indirectly to promote the patient's welfare and to guide those who have the responsibility for his care. For example, the rule requiring nurses to be in bed at a proper hour at night is designed primarily to safeguard the nurse's own health, but in spirit it extends to the welfare of the patient because it is well known that a nurse who has not had sufficient rest and sleep lowers her efficiency as a nurse, is more likely to make mistakes and the welfare of the patient suffers.

These rules do not prevent a spirit of helpfulness to each other; they do not hinder a nurse whose work is finished helping another who is delayed; they do prevent nurses from assuming responsibilities, and perhaps with the best of intentions, from doing harm. It may seem a small thing for a nurse to give a patient a glass of water, yet there are occasions when even a glass of water may be harmful to a patient, and for that reason she must go to those in charge of the patient and ask before doing it.

Rules and regulations in a hospital are the outgrowth of experience and conditions. They are a means of education and of promoting the comfort and general welfare of all connected with the hospital. Not every nurse in a hospital needs all the existing rules, but it is safe to say that unless conditions had arisen to make each rule necessary, it would not have been made. Instead of thinking of rules as irksome, they should be regarded as guideposts, necessary measures designed to promote the general good.

For Discussion

1. What is "ethics of nursing"?
2. What does a nurse owe to a patient?
3. Make a list of rules which nurses should observe in connection with patients.

2

HOSPITAL ATMOSPHERE

In all institutions there is that subtle, intangible thing called atmosphere. The nurse is affected by it, though often unconscious that she is being affected. The spirit or tone of the institution depends much on those in authority. Tone is the general character of the hospital as it relates to morals and manners.

It depends somewhat on the primary aims of the place. It depends greatly on the workers, the spirit which they put into their tasks, and their general mental attitude toward the work they have undertaken. In one hospital, professional courtesies are exchanged with doctors in a dignified way as they come and go. Patients' calls are responded to quickly and quietly. Doors are opened and closed noiselessly. No chattering is heard in corridors. There is an air of alertness and consideration for the patients' needs and of quiet dignity that gives a feeling of confidence in the nursing staff.

In another hospital, one hears nurses calling to each other in corridors, and flippant remarks about patients are overheard. Staff doctors are often heard talking in the corridors in the same tone they would use if going through a factory. But since nurses are more numerous and are very directly and constantly concerned with the comfort of the patient, they should be aware of the necessity of maintaining quietness in the sick room.

While the nurse is passing through the wards or attending classes, she is catching the influence of the personalities with whom she is associated, but she is not a passive individual. From the time she enters the hospital, she is impressing her ideals, standards, habits and personality on others. The individual nurse helps to create the atmosphere in which she works every day. The hospital will be made better or worse by her presence, by the way she does her work, by her daily conduct, on and off duty, by what she says, and by her general moral and spiritual influence. What she is, counts more than what she does.

There are numerous opportunities for friction and unpleasantness, which may react unfavorably on the patients. It is not necessary that probationers have to endure the snubbing that was so common years ago. They should not be regarded as unmitigated nuisances or scared by hearing all the weird and gruesome stories of hospital life. There are numerous little methods which a kindhearted, thoughtful nurse may use who has not forgotten the bewilderment and depression of the first few weeks of her probation period. No hospital can afford to have favorites, to grant certain nurses privileges to indulge in practices which it would forbid in others. The harmony and good feeling so desirable in a hospital must be based on equal justice for all.

The spirit of the nurse is revealed in a thousand different ways. Someone has said that one of the first and hardest lessons a nurse has to learn is to spell SELF with a little "s." It is often difficult for her to realize that success and advancement in this work, as in many others, usually comes to the one who continually studies how he may give his fellow being a little more, a little better service.

For Discussion

1. How may a nurse help in maintaining the right moral atmosphere in a hospital?
2. State several ways in which the spirit which a nurse manifests in everyday life may influence her success as a nurse.

3

LOYALTY

The patient is the most important person in the entire institution. He is the reason for its existence. His welfare and his comfort are and should always be given first consideration. Throughout a nurse's whole career, the patient's welfare should never be placed in the background of her thoughts or plans.

Loyalty to the patient's welfare demands, first of all, that his rights be respected and that his private affairs shall not be discussed with other patients or with people outside the hospital. Many centuries ago an ancient writer spoke of the tongue as an unruly member, and time has not changed its habits. A large part of the training for which a nurse must be responsible in herself is the training of her tongue, the cultivation in herself of refraining from discussing patients with outside nurses, with close friends and with members of one's own family or with any other individuals with whom a nurse associates, except those professionally concerned.

From the entrance of a nurse to the training school, she hears that her relations with patients must be "strictly professional" and she well knows the necessity of this rule. Yet there are nurses, many of them, who never seem to be able to keep their relations with patients within professional limits. They have a "confiding" way with them and before they have known their patients for twenty-four hours, they can be found relating their own private affairs which sick people should not be bothered with. Even love affairs are often unfolded to patients on a few hours acquaintance.

Nurses frequently think that they may tell anything they choose about their patients to their friends or family, or to other nurses. One foot of a newborn baby was slightly bent. A nurse told her friend that this baby had a club-foot. Of course, she thought her friend would not tell, but the story was quickly told and it spread to the circle of the patient's friends. Several friends came to the doctor to inquire if anything could be done for the club-feet of this baby. The story was eventually traced back to the nurse caring for the baby.

The nurse who has brought with her a predisposition to "tell things" which are better untold is one of the great problems of hospital life. How to deal with her, whether such nurses should be allowed to finish a nursing course, is one of the great unsettled questions. It rests entirely with the nurse herself whether she becomes this sort of problem in a hospital. She is the one who must learn to control her tongue. No one else can do it. Let her cultivate every day the habit of not telling things which need not be told, however great the temptation may be.

For Discussion

1. What limitations are needed when a nurse is asked information concerning a patient's condition?
2. What do you understand by the phrase, "loyalty to an institution?"
3. What is meant by professional conduct?

4

EVERYDAY ROUTINE

Nothing so tests character as the daily routine. We may be able to rise to sublime heights of courage and resourcefulness in times of emergency and yet easily fail to show the patience, tolerance, faithfulness and good judgment needed in the everyday routine. Every nurse is being tested in the everyday routine. Perfection is not expected, improvement is rightly expected.

One of the common failings of nurses is to neglect answering a call from one patient because they happen to be with another. There are few things more frequently complained of in regard to hospitals than the neglect to answer calls promptly. Nurses, in general, are too prone to excuse themselves on the plea of being "busy." We deal with human life, not with human bodies alone. No wonder those bodies rebel, now and then, and demand someone who recognizes their existence. It is important to develop the ability to attend to the wants of several patients and keep them all happy and satisfied, with no reasonable ground for feeling neglected. This calls for a spirit of cheerful readiness, which is quickly felt by patients and helps immensely in making them more willing to wait.

In the hospital it is essential that a nurse be systematic in her work, that she makes a careful division of her time between several patients, that she observes orders and regulations and develop a certain amount of speed in getting through her duties according to a prescribed method. The nurse will try to study how to systematize her work so that she gets through the day without being "rushed" in the last half hour.

All the time she is arranging her work she will be developing that quality called "executive ability" which is so much in demand. Ten nurses can follow orders, can do routine work well, if planned and directed by someone else, but one will be found who has developed the qualities of planning for others, of getting work done without needless fuss and friction. It is the nurse who has cultivated this quality who finds positions seeking her; she is in demand. Her services are worth more than those of the other nine.

Some standing rules for patients:

1. Be sure to speak a few reassuring words of comfort to patients as soon as possible after arrival.
2. Never ignore the existence of new patient until something has to be done for him.
3. Cultivate the habit of showing interest, and try to remember likes and dislikes when special points are mentioned.
4. Study how to be kind and thoughtful in seeking little things to be done for the patient's comfort.
5. Remember that we are dealing with afflicted souls, as well as afflicted bodies.

The nurse needs to remember that no education is ever secured without drudgery, and that all work, at times, seems to the doer of it as real drudgery. All nurses cannot be quick or brilliant. All cannot take the highest grade in examination, but all can be faithful, and there is no quality which means more to a nurse in meeting the stern tests of life, than the simple quality of being faithful to the trust reposed in one.

POWERS OF OBSERVATION

A nurse's efficiency is judged to a large degree by the extent to which she cultivates her power of observation and uses it in the daily routine. It is so easy to get into ruts in making records—noting only the routine things and failing to notice various important matters concerning patients. Many nurses follow the course of least resistance. It was the insistent habit of note-taking regarding the care of the sick that helped Florence Nightingale to lay the foundations for nursing as we have it today. If she had waited, as so many nurses do, to have every bit of knowledge administered by someone appointed for that purpose, if she had failed to see things all around her which bore on the things she was anxious to learn, she could never have accomplished the work she did. It should be the ambition of every nurse to gather up scattered bits of nursing knowledge and to cultivate to the fullest extent her observing powers concerning her patients.

For Discussion

1. What suggestions would you give a nurse in managing her morning work?

2. Mention one special quality in a nurse which largely determines her value as a worker.

3. Mention an important requirement in the care of the sick that was emphasized by Florence Nightingale.

5

HONESTY

In a hospital many questions of honesty and honor will present themselves to nurses—matters which they have never before had to consider. There is an ethical principle of right or wrong, involved in the smallest transaction. It is not always possible, nor should it be necessary for a nurse to have this pointed out to her by others. Pause long enough to ask whether she can justify herself in doing it whether she is being true to her best self in pursuing a certain course, whether she will lessen her own self respect by so doing. To be true to one's self, to one's own best ideals, is the hardest task a nurse will ever undertake.

Petty dishonesty is contagious, so is honesty. It remains for every nurse to decide which sort of influence she will exert. The most severe tests of character often come in the doing of routine duties. The practice of honesty enters every day into such matters as the taking of temperatures and of making records.

A nurse who was on duty had the care of the patients on one floor. A part of her duty was to take the temperatures of the children every morning. This became tedious. In many of the children there was little or no change in the temperature from morning to morning, so she decided to omit taking the temperatures of the children who showed little variation, and simply mark the charts each morning as though she had taken the temperatures. A nurse's records are an index to her real character, an everyday test of her honesty. It is of small comfort to know that the records looks well, are free from blots and erasures, etc., if they lie.

Strange as it may seem, the practice of common everyday honesty is the point at which many nurses fail. They apparently do not mean to be dishonest, but their consciences are either too undeveloped to perceive when a thing is honest or when it is dishonest, or they deliberately violate clearly accepted ethical principles of guidance that a child of ten ought to know. Occasionally, a nurse is found who has little or no regard for the rights and property of others. Such nurses will borrow, without asking, articles of clothing belonging to other nurses, wear them and loudly insist on the innocence of their intentions when called to account.

Mistakes may occur, but should be promptly confessed to those who have a right to know, and who are in a position to correct them. No nurse ever does deceive those in authority very long, though she may think she does. Honest confession of accidents or mistakes, whether intentional or unintentional, is one of the finest indications that a nurse can give that she is possessed of those high principles of conduct that should characterize a nurse.

For Discussion

1. Show how the principle of honesty enters into the taking of temperatures and the keeping of records.
2. In what way may a nurse's record keeping affect the general course of treatment prescribed for a patient?
3. What responsibility has a nurse who discovers that one of her associates is practicing dishonesty in her records
4. Is it dishonest to record a duty as done before it is done, when a nurse simply thinks she will do it?

5. If a nurse discovers that another nurse is administering sedative drugs without orders, what should she do? Has she any responsibility in the matter?

6

CARELESSNESS

Carelessness is a term having many shades of meaning. Webster defines it as "heedless; inattentive; unconcerned; unmindful; without thought or purpose; incautious; inconsiderate; remiss; not taking ordinary or proper care." Nurses are inclined to be either careful or careless before they ever see the inside of a training school. Part of the practice of carelessness is due to thoughtlessness; part of it is not knowing how the carelessness of one nurse, when multiplied by tens or hundreds, really affects the good work which a hospital is able to do for those who most need its help.

Most accidents occur not because the nurse is willfully careless, but because she is not sufficiently careful. She is willing to take a risk. It is this willingness to take risks, this neglect to use the precautions which have been taught, that results in many accidents for which nurses are responsible.

Occasionally, a serious accident occurs because a nurse did not understand the order, and this emphasizes the necessity of every nurse making sure that she understands what she is expected to do and how to do it. Too many accidents occur not because nurses cannot understand orders, but because they do not carefully read the orders, or because while they were reading the order they were thinking of something else.

Quite frequently, one very troublesome patient, who is making incessant calls on the nurse while she is trying to attend to other patients, will so confuse her mind that she neither thinks nor sees clearly, Excessive fatigue has the same effect. A tired mind affects working efficiency. This condition of confusion and exhaustion at the end of a day often results because a nurse "dawdled" over duties at the beginning, because she left till the end of the day duties which might have been done with ease several hours earlier.

Experience has shown that many accidents in the handling of drugs occur during the busiest hours when nurses are hurrying to get off duty at a given time. Experience has also taught that a nurse needs to be especially on guard at those hours. It is not real kindness in a nurse to cover up laxity or neglect in some other nurse. By covering up the results of careless habits we help a nurse to become more careless.

For Discussion

1. Give reasons why accidents are likely to happen in hospitals and why vigilance is needed to prevent their occurrence.
2. Describe 3 kinds of accidents to patients that you have observed, telling how each might have been prevented.
3. What should a nurse do when she discovers that she has given the wrong dose of medicine to a patient?
4. Why do accidents in the handling of drugs frequently occur?
5. Show how a nurse's mistake in arithmetic may cause the death of a patient.
6. State the precautions which you observe in giving medications.
7. Is a nurse responsible for accidents occurring if she had been told of necessary precautions but had not heeded what was taught her?

her opinions as to the disease a patient is suffering from.

To concentrate attention day in and day out on physical processes, without any attempt to go deeper into their meaning is to kill our sensitiveness to the other manifestations of life. If it were possible for nurses to separate the minds and souls of their patients from their bodies and nurse only the bodies, it would matter little what a nurse talked about in the presence of the sick, but since she is expected to minister to the whole patient, his mind as well as his body, it does matter a great deal whether the thoughts the nurse arouses in him are constructive or destructive in their influence over bodily functions.

An individual hears something that surprises or offends and the color of his skin changes; he blushes; capillary vessels in the face and neck dilate. The physical change has been directly due to the thought that came to his mind. We have seen people ready with a splendid appetite to partake a meal, when a disturbing bit of news arrives and at once the body loses its desire for food; the appetite has vanished.

A meal is eaten under the influence of distressing conditions, with anxiety filling the mind, and the glands that furnish the digestive fluid refuse to pour out their secretions; the food ferments, toxins are formed, and a train of miserable physical symptoms arise, if anxiety and worry continue.

We see a child who is hurt run to its mother, crying with pain. The mother kisses the spot, says a few comforting words; the mental state of the child has changed and the pain has gone. These illustrations might be multiplied to show what we all know to be true, that mental conditions powerfully affect bodily functions.

We may not fathom the deep secrets of psychology, but we do know that our own mental state is actively influenced by the people that we associate with. A friend with a happy optimistic temperament meets us, and he radiates the same feeling. He refuses to cherish gloomy forebodings, sees much that is good and beautiful in the world, maintains a quiet confidence and in some inexplicable way his attitude of mind is communicated to us. A fussy, nervous individual makes it impossible to get into a tranquil, restful state of mind while in his presence. Those who are well and active in the affairs of life are able to better resist such influences than are invalids who are shut in by the four walls of a sick room, and nurses should constantly remember that a good nurse ministers helpfully to the whole individual.

The possibilities of the power of thought are tremendous and no nurse can let this potent force in the sick room run riot. It is entirely within a nurse's power to refuse to harbor unpleasant thoughts, or to dwell on the sad and painful experiences of life. She can refrain from inflicting the story of her own unpleasant or harrowing experiences on a helpless patient who cannot escape from her presence.

Is it worthwhile to try and keep out of ruts in one's thinking and conversation? It is worthwhile for a nurse to try and improve her conversational standards? A good rule to start is with the following: "Whatsoever things are true, whatsoever things are lovely, whatsoever things are of good report; if there be any virtue, and if there be any praise, think on these things."

For Discussion

1. Mention common complaints that the public makes about graduate nurses?

2. What are several ways in which a nurse may help influence the mind of her patient and help to combat the depression of illness?

8
TACT

Tact is defined as the ready power of appreciating a situation, and of doing or saying that which is more suitable under the circumstances. It suggests the keenness of perception which enables a nurse to prevent awkward situations or to avoid difficulties arising from temperamental differences. The way in which a thing is told has so much to do with the way in which it is received, that all nurses need to study carefully the best way of putting disagreeable facts before a patient or his friends when asked for them, or when it is desirable for the facts to be known.

The untactful nurse always has a difficult time. She does not get along smoothly with people. There are sharp edges to her disposition. She may be conscientious and faithful, but her lack of tact prevents her from getting or keeping good positions or from making friends generally. She is very often called "self-opinionated" disposed to argue points when it really makes no difference, confident that she is right and that the patient or somebody else was wrong.

She creates trouble for people in authority by the inability to smooth out minor grievances of patients and prevent them from assuming larger proportions in the patient's mind. A spirit of genuine everyday kindness in a nurse is quickly felt by most patients, and one does not often find troubles arising for lack of tact, where the patient is convinced of the nurse's real desire and effort to be kind.

TACT AND THE PATIENT'S FRIENDS

In many cases the friends of patients make larger demands on us than the patients themselves. We are ready to make allowances for patients because of illness, but are often unwilling to make allowances for the mental suffering which a patient's friends are undergoing because of his illness. Quite often the father, mother, wife or husband of a much loved patient is suffering more deeply than the patient.

Perhaps the most difficult part of dealing with friends of a patient comes when rules have to be enforced. This is a point at which nurses need tact, judgment and also a good stiff spinal column. To keep one patient's visitor from annoying other patients is highly important, but when tactfully done it rarely offends. A discerning nurse will be able to see when some visitor is tiring the patient and will contrive to get rid of him whether the visitor's time limit has expired or not.

It is well to be guided to some extent in our dealings, not by the impression the friends make on us, but by the effect they have on the patient. A visitor may appear to us as a most unattractive and undesirable person. Her voice may be shrill, her habits noisy, and her appearance untidy. Yet to the patient she represents a familiar figure whose habits are unnoticed because of long familiarity with them and the effect on the patient may be good; his loneliness banished, he feels better.

For Discussion

1. Explain the term "tact'. How can it be cultivated?
2. How may an untactful nurse train herself to be tactful?
3. What attitude should a nurse present to a patient's friends?
4. Give some suggestions for a nurse in regard to the management of visitors, mentioning things to be avoided.

9

IMAGINATION

To see the real patient we must try to see him or imagine him in his natural environment; we must see him in relation to his family and associates, with whom he mingles in everyday life.

We see the patient in a free bed, or we think we see him. We think he should be profoundly grateful for all that is done for him. We frequently fail to appreciate how it must feel to some to become dependent on others; how it must fret a man or woman of independent spirit to be obliged to occupy a free bed.

In many cases an enforced stay, even a short one, in a hospital, means loss of wages, frequently debt, worry from fear of losing a job, anxiety over family problems, perhaps overdue rent, perhaps hungry children, all these and more. Yet in our short-sightedness, we know none of these things in the background, as we move in and out among the patients. We need not only good judgment but we need a kind heart and a mind that desires to understand the whole man, we need to see beyond the orders and general routine.

We may see a man who has struggled to make a small payment on a little home and what loss of work, what a stay in a hospital means in such a case. We may see a woman for whom the joy of life has been killed because of a wayward son or daughter or husband. In another, we may see one whose whole life has been a long struggle with adversity, for whom troubles have followed fast on each other, and who looks out into the future with dread and apprehension of what it may hold for her.

Would we be a little more patient, a little more kind, a little more attentive, if we could see back into their lives more clearly, and see each patient in his own setting, surrounded by the people and the things which make up his life?

The power to call up mental images, to modify our conceptions of things seen or felt, to combine different ideas so as to form new ideas in our mind has a large place in nursing. The lack of imagination is the cause of a very great deal of dissatisfaction where nurses are concerned.

Nowhere is the lack of tact or imagination likely to cause suffering then in the manner shown toward new patients. To the nurse, the new patient may be simply one more in the never ceasing procession of suffering or ailing individuals, one more bed or room occupied, one more to carry out standing orders for, one more name to go on the diet lists. To the patient, it is often a momentous experience in life, nearly always protested against and dreaded to some extent, nearly always fraught with anxiety, and more or less risk.

The nurse, who has trained her imagination so that she can at least dimly see things from the patient's viewpoint, will not come glibly into a patient's room and remark to a patient with a history of long standing pain "Is the pain gone this morning? She will try and remember the thousand and one little things that she would like done for herself if she occupied the patient's bed.

The nurse whose imagination is developed will not permit herself to smile or grow impatient where religious rites, ceremonies, or beliefs are concerned or mentioned. It is not uncommon to find nurses giggling or making remarks about religious obser-vances that were tremendously important to the patient. They did not imagine how the patient felt about it.

NOISE

What is the relation between a nurse's imagination and the noise that disturbs the sick so seriously? A very close relation, indeed! If a nurse had her imagination so trained that she could appreciate how noise jarred on sensitive nerves, would she be more careful, would she try to correct her noisy habits.

A list of the causes of preventable noises in hospitals would include: banging of doors, rattling of basins, noisy handling of chart files, moving of furniture, collecting of trays, etc. In nine cases out of ten the chief cause of noise, will be found to be the human voice.

For Discussion

Describe how the quality of imagination in a nurse may affect the comfort of her patients.

10
JUDGMENT

Good judgment comes only as the result of experience and of a wider knowledge than any nurse can hope to acquire in a short time. Many nurses fail to remember that the self-control, the power of wise decision, the resourcefulness, the quickening of the powers of observation and perception, the complete reliability which makes a good nurse a tower of strength have to be patiently acquired; they cannot be learned from books, cannot be put on with the uniform, they cannot be purchased. Nurses frequently come asking for a course of training when they do not desire training. They rebel against it. They would be satisfied with a moderate amount of instruction. They act as if they expected to have knowledge and judgment poured into them as though they were empty vessels.

JUDGING SEVERITY OF SYMPTOMS

The nurse may often have to judge the severity of a symptom of which the patient complains. Many patients are highly emotional and make a fuss out of all proportion to their condition. She will be open to the charge of harshness and indifference if she refuses to believe they are suffering and does not apparently try to relieve them. She may give such patients so much attention because they are noisy and trouble-some, that she neglects some silent sufferer who needs special attention. Then there will be the temptation to spend too much time with a patient who is congenial to her and to neglect others less congenial.

TRUTH-TELLING

It will be readily seen that truth-telling, even in the realm where others have the right to the truth, is a matter that requires much judgment and that the way the truth is told counts tremendously in its effects. Is truthfulness an absolute duty? Are we under obli-gation to tell the truth to anyone who chooses to ask it? We quickly learn that there are individual rights which should always be held precious.

When a patient who has the earliest recognizable signs of consumption asks, "Have I got consump-tion?" it would be conveying a false impression to say, "Yes, you have," and stop there. Ten to one his impression is that by consumption it means a disease invariable and rapidly fatal. To be true to the patient one must explain that what he means by consumption is the later stages of a neglected or unrecognized disease; that some people have as much trouble as he now has and get over it without finding it out; that with climate and hygienic treatment he has a good chance of recovery, etc. To tell him simply that he has consumption without adding any further explanation would convey an impression which in one sense is true. What is sometimes called the simple truth, the bald truth or the naked truth is often practically false. It needs to be explained, supplemented, and modified.

Proper nursing can be built only on a foundation of absolute truth as far as truth is known. The important question is not always, "Should I tell the truth or tell an untruth," but very often, "Is it necessary to tell anything at all at this time?" There is an old saying that "You are rarely sorry for the things you did not say."

CONFLICTS OF JUDGMENT

The spirit of intolerance with those whose opinions differ from ours is frequently seen. There are truths in the following quotation from a popular weekly paper which are worthy of consideration--lest we become self-opinionated, censorious, and uncharitable in our judgments of the motives of other workers who have every right to an opinion of their own.

"We are sometimes tempted into thinking that this would be a very much better and happier world if other folks would only agree with us and see things as we do. These conflicts of judgment and clash of opinions is not the bad thing that we sometimes take it to be. It is a way of progress. The radical who stirs up our inert conservatism may not be altogether agreeable to us, but we may need him just the same, and the man who opposes some of our pet plans and policies may be our good, though much disguised, friend. To agree to differ is sometimes much better than to agree. Conflicts of judgment will never cease, but contempt of other folks' judgment ought to. You are entitled to a point of view, but not to announce it as the center of the universe."

In dealing with the sick, or with the public, there are always at least two sides to every question that arises, and sometimes three or four sides. The nurse should avoid rushing to extremes; she should study to keep always an open mind before coming to conclusions.

For Discussion

1. If a nurse has favorites among her patients, giving special attention to one and "visiting"

with him while neglecting others, how should she be dealt with?

2. A nurse who has an unusual memory is able to pass written examinations taking a full 100% in many and a high grade in all. Her practical work is very inferior. She seems to lack judgment and tact and is not always truthful. What points should be considered? Give reasons for your answer.

3. How far should we speak the truth concerning patients?

11

THE NURSE HERSELF

The nurse's duty to herself should never be overlooked. It is just as real as her duty to others. Neither should it be given undue prominence. To have a proper sense of proportion, giving importance to certain things and placing less important things where they belong, is highly necessary for effective service. Since the nurse is the person to be trained, and since she will have a large part in the training of her own powers, it is very necessary that she make a careful study of herself, her possibilities, and her general make-up. She needs to know of some of the difficulties she is likely to encounter in the process of making a nurse out of very human material, which is a mixture of strength and weakness, of high and low impulses, striving for mastery.

CONSCIENCE

Among the fundamental requirements for the making of a good nurse we have placed the matter of conscience. As a state prisoner wrote, "Conscience is to the soul what health is to the body. No man knows what conscience is until he understands what solitude can teach him about it. As to the future, let us cast new resolutions to the winds; they are too often shallow and meaningless. Let us hear the inner voice that requires every man to mean well and to do his best in the world."

The nurse who enters a hospital for training comes or should come, with a conscious feeling that she must do right, that her purposes toward right conduct are fixed. It is expected that she has a fairly well-developed conscience which will help to guide her into right-doing. It influences her work, at every turn of the way, both in the hospital and in the great world outside. Taking reasonable health and intelligence for granted, the most important thing for a nurse to bring with her to school is a good conscience.

There is a very real relation between a nurse's conscience and infection, even though the subjects at first glance may seem wide apart. Her carelessness in health matters may easily create unnecessary burdens for those who are responsible for the nursing in the hospital. The nurse who neglects the hygienic precautions which she knows should be observed may easily carry infection from one patient to another, may add to the burden of sickness which they are already carrying, and may endanger life itself.

If a nurse has no sense of honor, nothing within herself that will keep her from doing small contemptible things, the greatest benefit that she can confer on the nursing profession is to leave it.

ANALYZING AN IDEAL

It is well, then at the beginning that a nurse should have a fairly clear idea of the kind of nurse she wishes to become. During the first year, before habits are too firmly fixed, there is excellent opportunity for any nurse to constantly endeavor to live up to the personal ideal she should keep before her.

Her ideals will grow and change with the passing years, but since she herself has a most important part in the training process, it is very desirable that she try and have a clear conception of the kind of nurse she is anxious to be. Let her think of the nurses she has known and read of, study the characteristics she admires in each, and also the characteristics which she thinks should be avoided. It is much better for the nurse to take a real person and try to analyze her habits and spirit than to frame a theoretical ideal which might not fit any woman who ever lived on earth, or in heaven.

What do you know of the illustrious founder of modern nursing, Florence Nightingale, of the qualities that made her great? What did she do in order to fit herself to improve nursing conditions? What difficulties did she encounter? What sort of woman was she, as a woman, apart from nursing? What do you most admire in her character? What nurses have you met whom you admired greatly, whom you wished to be like, and what was it that you admired? What qualities have you seen expressed in a nurses' life or conduct that you feel should be avoided or corrected?

AMBITION

Ambition is an eager desire for the attainment of certain objects is an important element in the making of a nurse, yet it may easily become an inordinate desire for honor, position, or power of some kind. Ambition is a quality which every individual should cultivate, yet diligently keep under control. It should help to carry a nurse forward to greater achievements, yet not at the expense of others. It cannot be too deeply impressed on a nurse that her own ambitions and ideals, the spirit which she puts into

chief determining factors in
great working world.

is that which leads a nurse to
ishes
erful   nd difficulties, rather than to
also   The man or woman who wins
ature   vels in working at, or working
and   others are ready to give up. It
hose   e nurse; it costs to be the finest
g or   and general attainments, along
the   se.
of a
e on

OF COURAGE

the   and alone, to meet opposition or
hat   being crushed, is a common cause
ies,   ise well-equipped women. They
nd   l someone to make up their mind
ws   ant questions, or to go ahead of
dy   he way. They are afraid to have
ew   any subject for fear of being
m   misjudged, or of meeting opposi-
ng   may fill a niche in the world;
he   ere is a place for them, but it is not
ht   t place.
st

PERSONALITY

Personality is that intangible thing that disting us from every other individual, exercises a po influence over the sick for whom we care, an over the well people with whom we associate. has endowed each of us with certain gif qualities and tendencies. The development o gifts and qualities which are good, the check correcting of tendencies that are detriment strengthening of our weak points, the cultivati pleasing personality, or the reverse, depends n the nurse herself than on anyone else.

Since the nurse will have a large part training of her own powers, it is very necessa she make a careful study of herself, her possib her general make-up. A nurse is successfu effective in her work not only by what she how to do, but by what she is. Call this psychology, if you will, but do not neglect i young women realize that learning how to p nursing duties is the smallest part of the tr process, that the drilling and disciplining woman inside the nurse, the development o character, and a right attitude of mind are th difficult parts in the making of a nurse.

TEMPER

Early in the training course the nurse learns that she must never argue with a patient; that she must learn to get along with others; that she must learn to control her temper. She knows or should know that the nurse who flies off in anger at trifles must acquire self-control, must master her feelings, or she will always be under a handicap as a nurse or as a worker in any line of activity.

Anger is usually looked on as a serious evil in life, yet anger has it place. The man or woman who can't get angry when occasion arises, who can't feel deeply indignant, is made of poor material. Yet it needs no argument to convince us that anger indulged in frequently or habitually is a sign of personal weakness, a sign that the individual has not learned to rule his own spirit, that he who indulges in anger hurts himself. The provocation many times will be great, yet the temptation to give vent to one's feeling in a snappy answer must be held in check.

What would the general atmosphere in a hospital if everyone followed the example of the nurse who, when busy with a bed patient, was asked by a patient in adjoining bed to give her a glass of water? Without stopping to think how it sounded or what the effect on the patient or ward would be, the nurse snapped out "Can't you see I'm busy? I haven't got 3 hands."

SELF CONTROL

Self control is the mental poise which enables you to scan guide posts and turns in the road without too much prejudice or predilection, with an open–mindedness that invites and recognizes reason. Self control keeps you from fighting, and keeps you from peace when fighting is needed. Self control wins many victories, but makes few enemies. And it is a great conserver of self-respect. It's not easy. It's hard. It's harder than controlling someone else. If you can control yourself you are doubly strong.

Self control means precisely what it reads—the full command of yourself, the captaincy over your mind and body under military discipline. It means to hold yourself in check when natural inclination unwisely lags. It is both a brake and throttle under your hand. Nurses need to cultivate the habit of not being easily excited.

Contact with suffering brings to a nurse a different sort of discipline. Every nurse needs to guard against allowing firmness to degenerate into hard heartedness; to be careful in developing endurance and self-control, that she does not lose some of the finer qualities which no nurse can afford to lose. We are with our fellow creatures in their hours of storm and stress when what is deepest and truest in them comes to light. Such contact is sure to affect us in one of two ways. It can ennoble us or it can make us callous. It is true she has to stand in the shadows with those who are in trouble, but her face can always be turned toward the sun, so that the true light may not only enable her to see her duty, but may beautify it.

The expression of the face, the tone of voice, and the character of our touch all affect the patient's comfort and condition. The patient who is anxious about his condition will study carefully the expression of the face of doctor or nurse to see if he can discern from the face what the opinion is which they do not openly express in words.

Therefore, controlling the expression of the face and of the voice, so that neither face nor voice expresses anxiety, alarm or surprise, however serious the occasion, is one of the important lessons a nurse must learn. Tone and manner often convey more than the spoken word. It is, however, not necessary or desirable to always repress the expression of pleasure or gladness, either in face or voice, when all is going well. A happy quality of optimism in a nurse is an element much to be desired and it can be cultivated.

THE VOICE

The quality of the voice may seem to a nurse something which she cannot control, something with which she was born and for which she is not responsible, yet a little thought and study of herself will convince her that habit has much to do with it. A nurse may be habitually loud-voiced or gentle-voiced when she enters the school and may never have had attention called to it. She must train herself to realize that her habits of voice influence greatly the comfort of the patients and also their appreciation of her value as a nurse. It is hard to imagine the amount of unnecessary discomfort that the sick are obliged to suffer because of the undisciplined voice in nurses and because of the thoughtless chatter that is so often heard in corridors.

Study your own voice. Do you speak distinctly, firmly, yet gently, or do you drawl your words out as if you had no energy behind them? Is your voice, or habit of speaking, harsh, discordant or unnecessarily loud? Is your tone quick, sharp, shrill has it that piercing quality which jars sensitive nerves and often causes real pain? Do you mumble your words or speak in whispers? Do your tones indicate a cheerful, kindly disposition or the opposite? Have your tones that quiet, gentle, firm note of authority and strength which inspires confidence?

TOUCH AND MOVEMENT

Few defects in a nurse are more quickly noted by patients or observers than the lack of gentleness. A nervous, self-conscious nurse often jars the bed and the patient, slams doors, and drops things. This is excusable at the beginning. It becomes a serious defect if it continues. By our touch, we may convey to the patient our feeling of sympathy and tenderness, our appreciation of his weakened condition, our desire to be helpful. We reveal our character in our touch, to a considerable extent. The human hand has in it a wonderful power to soothe. However, it can easily be used in such a way to indicate familiarity of manner against which a nurse needs to guard with all patients.

Habits to be avoided are a careless attitude in standing as if the backbone were weak and needed support; a lounging posture in sitting; leaning against the bed or other support; sitting on the patient's bed.

GOOD MANNERS

It is in the daily 'hussel and bussel' of hospital life to remember and practice the grace of courtesy. The time goes so fast, interruptions are numerous, and there are so many duties to claim our attention that almost before we know it the staccato note has crept into our voice, and we are nothing if not abrupt. Thronging duties hem us in on every side until sometimes the common courtesies of life are allowed to slip from us–people are deaf, people are stupid. Yet some of the busiest people have been noted for their good manners, while those possessed of ample leisure are not always the most courteous.

Nurses are mistaken when they regard themselves as isolated units or when they try to deceive themselves into thinking that their manners or methods affect only themselves. The nurse who is sullen, defiant when she is shown her mistakes and what she must do to correct them, constitutes a real problem in every school. Too often, instead of accepting rebuke, she goes about clamoring for sympathy, proclaiming to other nurses that she is tired of being scolded or that someone has picked on her and indulges in self-pity that is always unwholesome.

Good manners are not incompatible with sincerity. Nearly always there is something pleasant to say if we will only say it, which is infinitely more acceptable than the abrupt word or unsmiling look.

Courtesy establishes friendly relations at once and goes far to oil the wheels of daily life.

Surely, if any members of the community ought to cultivate good manners, nurses should do so. At the very commencement of her career a well-mannered girl stands on a different footing from her more uncouth companion. Her fellow nurses like her, the patients take to her, the head nurse sees in her a promising pupil. As she goes on, she finds difficulties smoothed by her invariable courtesy; she can bend patients, even members of committees yield to her charm of manner.

A nurse's manner reflects, to a degree, her inner qualities. Two things which go far toward making a good impression are a sincere interest in the patient, not a feigned interest or "case" interest and a spirit of genuine kindness that finds its expression in numerous ways. A nurse who is genuinely kind will find that virtue covers up a multitude of other defects.

For Discussion

1. What do you mean by the term, "personality"? In what way does it influence a nurse's success? Does a nurse have any control over her personality?

2. Is there such a thing as righteous anger? Give an example. What place has anger in dealing with patients?

3. What is conscience? What effect does it have on the life and work of a nurse?

4. How may a nurse's voice affect the comfort of patients?

5. State why you believe self-control is indispensable to a nurse.

6. What qualities of voice should a nurse cultivate? What qualities should be avoided?

7. Show how touch, movement and manner of walking may reveal character.

8. Mention 3 qualities of movement which nurses should try to cultivate.

9. Describe the nurse you have met who came nearest to your ideal.

10. Mention several ways in which the expression of a nurse's face may affect the attitude of the patient.

11. Mention any quality which seems to you a substitute for courage. How is courage acquired?

12. What is meant by the phrase, "the courage of one's convictions"?

13. Why is it that some nurses have convictions and others do not? How much does one's early training have to do with convictions?

14. If a nurse is lacking in ambition to the responsibilities or demands of a position, what can be done to make her a success?

15. What is callousness in nursing? What daily preventive measures would you recommend a nurse to use?

12

Types of Nurses

The young woman who enters training school for nurses finds that it is an entrance into a new world — a world having laws and customs differing widely in many respects from those of the world outside. She finds that the science and art of nursing is inseparably bound up with the science and practice of moral conduct and that one phase of training influences the other every step of the way. Many "diamonds in the rough" are admitted for training in the hope that, through training, the fine qualities that are believed to be in them may be developed and the rough edges smoothed away. This process takes time and patience.

In every school there are nurses who seem to have no higher motive than simply to secure a diploma, and who wish to do as little as possible and study as little as they can possible manage to get through; who seem to be in no way desirous of correcting glaring defects in character, even when attention is called to them. Others are quick but superficial, content to slight their duties whenever it seems convenient and have no aspirations toward thoroughness.

It is the nurse who after having her attention called to the need of improvement yet shows no sign of improvement, no effort to correct the fault or weakness is a big problem in many a school. Her technical work may be good, her disposition most deplorable. She may be tolerated and allowed to finish her course because she commits no open or flagrant misdemeanor to justify her dismissal.

Another type is slow in grasping new ideas and methods, but makes up for this in their faithfulness to details and their loyalty to the patients. They quickly develop the quality of being dependable and impart a feeling of security and confidence when they are at work.

The nurse who is unwilling to study or sacrifice, who comes to the hospital "to see if she will like it" who feels that social pleasures or her engagements should take precedence to duty, needs either to change her attitude of mind or to choose some other line of work that will leave her free to make social engagements and do as she pleases with her time. She does not desire to be a nurse strongly enough to pay the price cheerfully.

The stony manner so frequently used in portraying nurse characters is unfortunately not entirely an imaginary quality. It exists in far too many nurses. Constant daily associations with strangers tend to make some silent, unresponsive, unsympathetic. They go about their business self-contained and indifferent to others. They ask but little of others and never go out of their way to do an unasked kindness to anyone. Most people intend to be kind, and are willing to be kind, provided they happen to think about it, but the trouble with nurses as with many other people is that they often fail to perceive an opportunity to show personal kindness to a stranger. They may be of sterling worth under this hard crust, but their better qualities seldom find their way to the surface. These people sometimes become embittered because their good qualities and real ability remain unrecognized, while others less reliable and not half as clever, easily win promotion or praise.

Another group of nurses demonstrate quickly their power of constructive thinking and planning. They manifest that quality known as "initiative." They see things to be done and do not have to be told every slight detail. They see things out of place and put them where they belong, without waiting to be told. They are not given to wasting time in gossip and get along well with their associates.

The grumbling nurse is found at some time in all schools. She may be capable, and of more than average intelligence, but she is unable to adapt herself to the rules and restrictions. Such nurses grumble about rules, work, food hours, till they succeed in keeping all with whom they associate uncomfortable. The habit of grumbling in some people is chronic and usually it is to a greater or lesser degree contagious. There is only one thing to be done in regard to a nurse of this type, who persists in grumbling and stirring up discord that poisons the atmosphere of the place, and that is to get rid of her.

A REAL GRIEVANCE

The nurse with a real grievance belongs to a different class. That, even in this twentieth century, nurses sometimes suffer from unnecessary and preventable discomfort, cannot be denied.

Very rarely is anything gained by airing one's grievances in corridors and bedrooms, with those who are in no position to correct conditions. First, be sure it is a real grievance and not a fancied one. Second, write a statement of the grievance on paper, and let it cool for a few days, or longer. Be sure it is not exaggerated. If it still seems a real grievance that can be and should be remedied, go to the person in authority, who is in a position to correct the conditions complained of and see if something may be done to improve matters.

For Discussion

1. Make a list of faults you have observed in a nurse which you think all nurses should avoid.
2. Describe some other types of nurse who you know—nurses who will not fit into any of the types mentioned.

13

THE NURSE'S HEALTH

A nurse's health is her most important asset. Every nurse has a physical, mental, spiritual, and social side, all needing care and cultivation. However skillful she may be in her profession, she cannot hope to attain her highest success in any line of nursing activities if she is in a debilitated, uncertain condition of health.

In every class of probationers there are likely to be found three types of nurses:

1. Those who give up and go to bed for very slight and sometimes fancied ailments.

2. Those who will persistently assert that they are not ill and who remain on duty when their own common sense tells them they should be in bed.

3. Those who take a sensible middle ground and when they do not feel as well as usual, frankly come and report the matter to those in charge, realizing slight indisposition, if attended to promptly, may prevent suffering and loss of

time to the nurse herself and inconvenience to those who have to assume her duties if she has to be sent to bed.

HANDS AND FEET

Two very important parts of a nurse's anatomy which need careful guarding to keep them in good condition are her hands and her feet. Under the finger nails is a favorite lurking place for germs and the careless nurse, however good her intentions, may easily carry infection in her own body as well as infect others. Careful cleansing of the hands before meals or before partaking of food of any kind is a rule that cannot be too closely observed. Soap and water applied to the hands freely and frequently are powerful safeguards to the health of a nurse. Breaks in the skin of the hand, hang nails, minor cuts, etc., should be carefully attended to, as they afford an avenue for the entrance of infectious germs to the body.

Since much of a nurse's work requires standing or walking, the condition of the feet is of prime importance. Most schools require a nurse to bring with her a pair of comfortable, well-fitting shoes with low heels. A few schools have the feet of all nurses examined and special shoes prescribed. Apart entirely from the matter of comfort, which is highly important, it is plain that no nurse is at her best, nor in condition to do her best for her patient, if she is suffering tortures from tight, badly fitting or unsuitable shoes.

SLEEP

The temptation to violate the rule which requires nurses to be in bed between certain hours comes to most nurses, yet both she and the patients suffer if a nurse fails to get the sleep required. If a nurse is unable to sleep after she has used all the measures she knows, perhaps a nurse is indulging in strong tea or coffee just before retiring; perhaps the room she sleeps in is not well ventilated or darkened; perhaps there are house noises. In any case, since a nurse cannot do her best work without a reasonable amount of sleep, it is important that everything possible be done to help her. Remember that fatigue has an important effect on the channels along which our impulses travel, with the natural result of weakening the resistance of the will. A prolonged condition of fatigue is thus a source of great danger. To the tired brain, facts appear distorted. Values are displaced, sanctions are ignored, resolutions are forgotten, good intentions fly to the winds. A wise rule is never make an important decision when one is physically or mentally weary or depressed or not in good condition physically.

SOLITUDE

Every individual needs solitude, apart from the distractions of life and away from the influence of other minds. This time of solitude a nurse will rarely get unless she insists on it. Much time is wasted by nurses in off-duty hours by aimless gossiping about the incidents of the day, gossip which may be harmful to the nurse, even if not malicious.

SUNSHINE

Outdoor recreation, taken some time during the hours of sunshine, is imperative if general vitality is to be kept up. Sunshine is a great vitalizer and restorer. It increases our power to resist disease, quiets irritated nerves, and keeps us sweet tempered and at our best.

DIET

It is along dietary lines that nurses err more frequently than anywhere else in matters of health. Too free indulgence in tea or coffee, nibbling at candy, cake, nuts, etc., in off duty hours, night suppers in rooms are common causes of ill health among nurses in training.

OVERSTRAIN IN NURSES

Overstrain in nurses with the resultant loss of equilibrium and disturbance of nerve balance, is usually due to a combination of causes. Loss of sleep, insufficient exercise in the open air, digestive difficulties–these combined with worry, are found to a greater or less degree in most cases. All nurses suffer from overstrain in the early weeks of their training, due to the mental and physical effort required in getting accustomed to new surroundings and duties, in trying to remember the multiplicity of new things that need to be grasped in the very beginning. The period of overstrain passes away in a short time, and the nurse develops a higher degree of resistive power and endurance in much the same way that an athlete develops muscular strength and skill.

WORRY

Worry plays a much greater part in sapping the vitality than any other cause. It is a veritable demon that robs life and work of its joys, poisons the nervous organism at its very centers, and affects the smooth harmonious working of the machinery of the body in a variety of ways. If efforts are not made to combat it, worry soon becomes a habit that lessens efficiency and reacts adversely on the nurse. A good holiday is often the best antidote for worry.

Dr. J. H. Kellogg gives the following rules for those who would cure themselves of worry: "To cure worry you must cultivate hope; to cure pessimism you must deliberately cultivate optimism. You must force your mind into optimistic channels of thought. This can best be accomplished by reading optimistic authors and talking with optimistic people. It is a well-known fact that the best actors often actually experience the emotions which they depict in their acting. When counterfeiting laughter, for instance, they often actually experience the thrill of good cheer which normally accompanies the act of laughing. It one feels disagreeable and sullen, he may dissipate the spell by assuming an air of cheerful amiability and sociability quite different from the inward feeling, with the result that the mask of geniality will soon permeate the mind and character."

RECREATION

Inseparably interwoven with health is the subject of recreation. Nurses in training and after training, often show a lack of good sense in regard to how they spend their off-duty periods and holidays. True recreation is a combination of things; change of air, getting completely away from the hospital or one's work; change of thought, the banishing for the time everything connected with nursing; and change of exercise and habits.

It is just as much a nurse's duty to learn to rest properly and wisely as it is to learn right methods of work. A proper amount of sleep and rest are a necessary part of recreation. In her efforts to secure what she thinks is recreation, a nurse too often becomes unwisely fatigued, and return to her work and studies worn out rather than refreshed. Tiresome shopping expeditions are planned; errands are undertaken for other people; exhausting excursions are taken; late hours are indulged; or perhaps, week after week, the nurse frequents moving picture shows in her afternoon off duty.

Shorter and more frequent periods of rest yield better results, as a rule, than longer vacations. It is often difficult to make a nurse believe that what she wants in regard to vacation is not always best.

FRIENDSHIP

The nurse who desires to maintain a true balance in her life, will find that the friendships she forms during training will have much to do with the progress that she makes in various directions. For a nurse in training her most wholesome friendships will usually be made with those of her own class. Friends have much to do with the making or marring of both a nurse's happiness and reputation. They both reflect her character and profoundly affect it. A mistake which many nurses make is the formation of friendships on very short acquaintance, and with whom they have but a superficial knowledge. Another mistake is that of allowing the feeling to develop that one's friend is an absolute necessity to one's happiness. It is a mistake to attach one's self to one person so exclusively that one neglects to make other friends who might mean much in one's life.

The realization that there are people in life who will pose as friends, because in some way an individual is useful to them, and who will drop him as soon as the novelty wears off and they meet another who seems for the moment more attractive or useful, comes to many nurses as one of the bitter experiences of life; but it is by such an experience that one learns to be cautious in the choice of friends. It is neither wise not necessary for nurses to cut themselves off from all social life; they need friends — friends and acquaintances who are not of the world of sickness in which they live. The elements of friendship are hard to analyze, but one thing is certain, that real friendship is always unselfish.

A few sensible health laws: To eat well, neither too much nor too little and of proper food; to play often; to laugh; to think much of others and little of one's self; to spend a part of every day in the open air; to be hopeful; to look on the bright side of life; to have always some work to do, some responsibility to carry and whatever happens, to be good-natured.

For Discussion

1. Can you trace any relationship between ethics and health as it relates to nursing?
2. Outline some precautions which nurses should use in the care of their hands and feet.
3. What suggestions would you give to a nurse who wished to keep at her maximum health?
4. Make a list of rules of health which you have seen nurses violate.
5. Mention some causes of overstrain in nurses.

6. What is the effect of worry on digestion, on the power to sleep, on the general health?

7. When worry seems to be settling into a habit, what can or should an individual do to combat it?

8. Mention several ways in which you have observed that nurses do not use good judgment in regard to recreation.

9. In the matter of recreation, what 3 things would you suggest that a nurse try to do, what 3 things to avoid?

10. How many true close friends is an individual likely to have at one time?

11. Mention some things which a nurse must do if she desires to have a circle of friends.

12. What are some of the perils of friendship in hospital life?

13. Give several reasons why a nurse needs to cultivate friendships among people who are not in any way connected with the world of sickness.

14

DEVELOPING A SYMMETRICAL LIFE

Apart from obtaining a nursing education and experience, every nurse is developing a life. To direct and develop this life with a wholesome outlook on the world depends on the nurse whether she accomplishes this or not. The possibilities of becoming warped and stunted in growth, of becoming one-sided and narrow, are present in every nurse's life. No nurse is doing justice to herself who does not ally with some great movement to help her to keep a proper balance in her life. There are, perhaps, no reminders which nurses, as a body, need more frequently than that they should try to see both sides of a question before coming to conclusions; that they should study to keep always an open mind, and avoid letting petty prejudices possess them. If one is to successfully accomplish this, one must cultivate acquaintance with "many men of many minds." There is found in the person who is "broad" in his viewpoint of life, a geniality, and generosity that gives to him a genuine charm of character.

THE VALUE OF NEW INTERESTS

A variety of interests in life helps greatly to form a just estimate of relations and values. It is said of certain women that they knew of no great events to talk about, so they talked about small things as if they were great. Many nurses indulge in gossiping, endlessly, about their patients, at meals, in bedrooms, on street cars, and in public places, simply because they refuse to make the effort to direct their conversation into other channels of thought. Beyond all this, there is found the person who has read widely and is well informed.

To the man or woman who has allowed himself or herself to become engrossed with one interest, or has allowed one cause to loom up and fill the whole horizon, there is a constant temptation to go to harmful extremes, and to regard those who have more varied interests in life and a different viewpoint as enemies to the cause they have at heart. Fifteen minutes a day or less spent in scanning events in the daily papers will serve to keep a nurse posted as to the progress of the important developments in her own community and country and keep up a wholesome interest in the world outside. An hour a week with magazines which give a review of world progress will wonderfully widen a nurse's outlook on life.

Membership in a nurses' association should help to combat the perils of narrowness which threaten every nurse. It should give a view of national movements, and an opportunity to cooperate in many of the broader programs and efforts for human betterment. There is a real danger of a nurse joining so many nursing associations that she does not count for much in any of them. There is also the danger of becoming so engrossed in nursing affairs that one has neither time nor energy left to give to any other good movements. Nurses who commit the blunder in thinking of nursing exclusively cannot fail to grow narrow in their views.

One of the easiest and most natural ways that a nurse can keep out of the ruts of monotony in thought and conversation is to maintain her relationship with some church, attend its services as regularly as possible and try to keep in touch with what her own church is doing at home and on foreign fields. The religious spirit is one that can't be hurt, shocked or wounded. Failure does not seem to touch the religious man. Such a person gives great calm and happiness, can't but be enthusiastic, because he is always finding what is surprising and fresh; fresh meaning, fresh value in the old, fresh opportunity and experience in the new. Such a person is everybody's friend because he finds everybody interesting.

Ye Have Need of Patience. It is a common failing of nurses as of many other workers, that they clamor for immediate benefits or results from some organization with which they have allied themselves. If these benefits are not speedily forthcoming they lose interest. Many of the results which accrue from organizations are indirect, and a nurse very often benefits in proportion to the amount of herself that she puts into it. "Learn to labor and wait" is an admonition frequently needed in this age when the tendency is to expect to reap a harvest before a seed has had the time to germinate and really take root.

Whatever other organizations a nurse belongs to, she should endeavor to become a member of at least one organization in which men and women are working together toward a common end. The masculine viewpoint on many problems is well worth having; in many circumstances it is essential to a well-balanced judgment. Better social and community conditions are only secured as men and women work together. The millennium will not be ushered in by women alone, or by men alone, but by men and women working together.

For Discussion

1. Of what value to nurses are varied interests in life?
2. Show how a variety of interests tends to strengthen character.

15

AFTER GRADUATION

What shall I do after graduation? How and where shall I use the training I have acquired? Where does duty lie when one ventures beyond training school? What should the individual nurse's aim be as she leaves the school?

It is well for a nurse to have a dual aim in view, an immediate or present aim and an ultimate aim, something ahead to strive to reach. It is not well for her to be too positive at first about what she will or will not do. The path of duty is rarely clearly marked out very far ahead. We advance step by step. We live one day at a time. We do not need to see tomorrow's duty. We do not know what opportunity is going to offer us. We do know that experience as an independent worker is necessary, and a valuable asset. The opportunity most coveted will rarely be waiting for a nurse as she leaves the school, but the lesser opportunity which may prove the first step toward it will probably present itself in due time.

To do good work in any nursing field, it requires that a nurse must have, besides her technical training, some enthusiasm, adaptability, and liking for the work. Occasionally one meets the unusual nurse, the nurse who apparently can follow any one of several different lines of work and appear to do well in all of them. Such nurses have probably acquired, before and after coming to school, a variety of experiences and education along different lines that serves to supplement their nursing training.

The majority of nurses cannot do two or three kinds of work equally well. The difficulty with many nurses is that they become hopeless drifters, rarely staying at any one thing long enough to become really proficient, never being able to say of any one kind of work, "this is where I feel I can do the best work" or "I have found my work." Very often, a certain form of nursing has been idealized in the nurse's mind. She sees it from a distance, and it appears to have a halo around it. She may be honestly convinced that such work, above of all others in the world, is for her. A bit of experience is then her greatest necessity.

There are disagreeable features in all branches of work, including nursing, and each has it compensations. There is such a thing, however, as "working against the grain", working in conditions which are singularly distasteful and it is certain that one's best work will not be accomplished in such circumstances. There is an excess of nervous energy expended where one is working against one's natural bent, where there is friction, and where one feels there is not the best use of one's powers. In time this reacts adversely on the health of the worker.

It makes little difference how capable and skilled a nurse may have become during her training, if she is not willing to work; if she is continually looking out for the easiest cases and places and refusing those which would probably mean serious or hard work, she can never be a successful nurse. Quite frequently a nurse who is a habitual shirker may be able to get through school because someone constantly supervised her and kept her up to the mark, but when she becomes an independent worker, her habitually lazy habits reassert themselves. This type of nurse does more to create prejudice against nurses than any other type.

If a nurse desires a life that is abundant, rich, and satisfying, yielding a full measure of happiness, she will find it through service, and in no other way. The law of happiness is based on social service, or service to society, to others. Had Florence Nightingale sought her own happiness and convenience, had she planned for herself a life of ease, she would never have carved for herself a niche in the most enduring temples of fame—the hearts of the people.

ADAPTABILITY

The nurse who lacks adaptability "fusses" when she cannot have her own way, is unable to see a situation from the viewpoint of others, is unable or unwilling to concede to others rights which she demands for herself. Her own convenience and comfort are usually uppermost in her mind, though she would be the last to admit it. The chief difficulty lies in the unwillingness to recognize her own defects and limitations or the reasons for her failures. She too frequently suffers from what Florence Nightingale termed "the vice of self-sufficiency." She does not make a real effort to "fit into" the varying situations in which she finds herself, so there is constant friction. She may be a capable nurse but "hard to get along with." Florence Nightingale deplored the fact that nurses were more anxious for positions than they were to find out what the positions were desiring in them and how near or how far they came from meeting the expectations of those who employed them.

FIRST IMPRESSIONS

First impressions apply to obtaining a desired position. The wearing of much jewelry and a lingerie blouse cut indecently low in the neck has prevented a nurse from a coveted position in an institution. The superintendent decided that the jewelry was unnecessary for nurses and indicated personal vanity, and the indecently low-cut blouse suggested that its wearer would not be a good example to nurses.

The failure to keep an appointment made for a certain hour has often settled the question of the desirability of a nurse for some positions. She was unbusiness-like and was likely to fail in various other directions. A nurse's word should mean something if she ever hope to attain to any position of trust. If she agrees to go to a certain place at a certain time, she should be there unless some accident befalls her, or she should notify in time those who are depending on her or expecting her that she cannot keep the engagement.

A good impression of self confidence is important. This must be guarded that it shall not become conceit which always offends and antagonizes. If you do not have a good opinion of yourself, how are you going to impress others that you are worthy of their good opinion? A woman who is willing and knows that she can do good work is likely to be given an opportunity to do it.

THE NEED TO STUDY

The quality of being teachable is one of the most important that a nurse has to cultivate, not only at the beginning, but all through her nursing career. In the beginning, a nurse does not need to know everything about nursing; the important thing is whether she is capable of learning and eager to do so.

Conferences and meetings with social service and charity workers are always broadening and educative. There are many points at which the work of the nurse and the social service worker touch, and it is important that a nurse be able to appreciate the work and the viewpoint of social workers who are making large contributions to state and community betterment.

To fill positions well requires that a nurse must be ready every year or two to take up some kind of study. The nurse who neglects or refuses to study, soon falls behind. As long as she is working, a nurse should expect to be a student. She should invest in books and magazines as a mechanic does in tools that she may keep abreast with the march of modern progress.

For Discussion

1. Give some reasons why rings and other jewelry are out of place on a nurse.

2. Discuss what you consider is the right attitude of the nurse at graduation toward the needs of the world and the problems that confront her.

3. What do you understand about adaptability and how is it cultivated? Show why it is important in a nurse's success.

4. Give some suggestions to a nurse who desires to make a good first impression.

5. State some important things which a nurse should consider before making a choice of any area of nursing.

6. Give some reasons why a nurse should not settle down close to the hospital in which they were trained.

16

THE HEAD NURSE

The head nurse's position is one of increasing importance in hospital and nursing life. It offers the graduate opportunities to secure executive experience. The nurse who has proven successful as a head nurse will find many other doors of opportunity awaiting her.

Thus far little attempt has been made to provide a special course for head nurses that would help them to better understand their place in hospital activities. There is not and never can be a fixed code of ethics for her. She will always have to learn much by experience and observation; but there are certain fundamental principles in ethics which pertain especially to the head nurse—principles which affect so vitally the harmony and tone and comfort of the whole institution.

The quality of fairness is one which every successful head nurse should try to possess. It must be one of the foundation stones in her system of management, to be lived up to whether it is easy or difficult.

It is natural to like some patients, doctors or nurses better than others, but justice should keep an executive from allowing her likes and dislikes to influence her management. Favoritism in any way leads to trouble.

The fine art of finding fault pleasantly is one which every head nurse must cultivate. Much of her work must consist of correction and the way in which this is done will have much to do with good feeling and harmony. No really successful head nurse will allow herself to administer reproofs in the presence of others. This is always resented. To be able to administer rebuke without arousing antagonism is a quality which must be given diligent cultivation. There is plenty of opportunity to practice this particular virtue.

Seeing beneath the surface is another quality which head nurses need to develop. Minor failures and errors are to be expected of nurses, and while they are not to be overlooked, it is necessary that an effort be made to look beneath the surface and appreciate the spirit which was behind the failure. It takes no special amount of genius or skill to find fault. It takes skill to be able to give constructive suggestions that will help to correct known faults.

Appreciation of work well done and of general improvement is an important habit for the head nurse to cultivate. There are but few individuals who will keep up sustained effort to improve, if nobody cares or seems to notice. Careless thinking and practice in nurses can often be traced to lack of appreciation of their best efforts.

Progressiveness and ambition are always found in the successful head nurse. She is constantly looking about for methods which will add to the efficiency of her department. The head nurse's point of view has much to do with the smooth running of hospital machinery. To be successful she must be able to see, to some extent at least, the needs of the institution as a whole, and to adapt herself to those needs without comment on particular situations. Failure to do this is a sign of unfitness for the work, or for greater responsibilities.

Another phase of unprofessional conduct is shown in lack of respect for authority. No one is fitted to command who has not learned to obey without grumbling. This was one of the principles laid down by Florence Nightingale — the nurse who is fitted for the responsibility of directing others must observe rules made for the good of all and must respect the wishes of those in authority over her. No nurse who is really fitted for head nurse responsibility will wish or try to be a law unto herself.

TEACHING QUALITIES

The new conception which is being forced on nurses by the demands of the age is that she is not only a supervisor and executive, but a teacher who has exceptional opportunities to teach much of practical value which will never be taught, unless she measures up to her opportunity. While this new conception makes more demands on the nurse it has in it great possibilities for the development of the head nurse's own powers. Certainly the head nurse should be satisfied with nothing but the highest standard of life and conduct for herself. Next to experience, the best of all teachers for nursing is a good example.

This is a point at which many good head nurses seem timid. There is one thing to have a certain kind of knowledge and a different thing to impart it effectively. There is a current belief that teaching instinct is born with an individual, that teachers as well as nurses "are born, not made." To some extent this may be true, but it would surprise most people if they really knew how much thought, study and effort the supposed "born teacher" had put forth to reach a stage of proficiency. There is usually a vast difference between what the individual was by native endowment, and what she has become by the study of the art of imparting knowledge.

First among the teaching qualities which the head nurse should cultivate is how to utilize the teaching opportunities of her department. She needs to study how to tie up the theoretical teaching which a nurse has received, to ward work.

Repetition is an important element in successful teaching. We learn that the pupil is not always to blame because she did not retain the thing we thought we had taught her. Perhaps we did not make the point quite clear, and did not properly emphasize it. Patience with the slow pupil is another quality which head nurses need to cultivate.

The art of questioning occupies a most important place in teaching. The success and efficiency of our teaching depends more on the skill and judgment with which we put questions than on any other single method used in theoretical teaching.

For Discussion

1. Explain why the head nurse is such an important factor in hospital life.

2. What offers the greater possibilities of development to the head nurse herself?

17

A NURSE AND HER MONEY

An important indication of character is the way an individual spends the money he earns. The charge that nurses are unbusinesslike in their habits, inclined to extravagance, apt to live up to the extent of their incomes, is frequently made and with some degree of truth.

Five Pertinent Questions for a Woman earning a Salary

1. How much have I earned in my life?
2. How much could I have saved?
3. How much do I possess free and clear now?
4. How much of the difference between earnings and possessions has been frittered away?
5. What am I going to do from this time on to secure my living expenses in sickness and in old age?

In the study of ethics, it is certain that the right or the wise use of money should not be overlooked. It is also certain that it is easier to earn money than to spend it wisely, that the wise investment of the reward of one's own labor is one of the big problems of life. Whether one is considering the spending of one dollar or one thousand, the matter is an investment.

To a great many young nurses, $25 a week seems a large sum, and in the first flush of elation over their wage-earning ability, they proceed to invest in various items of longed for finery, and presently when work is slack they find themselves with no bank account, a very slim pocketbook, and expenses going steadily on. Borrowing small sums of money from other nurses is certain to create difficulties for the one who borrows and for the one who loans. It is no disgrace to have to borrow money, but the things for which nurses borrow money are often exceedingly ridiculous. There are dignified and proper ways of securing such loans without embarrassing one's associates by asking for the loan of money.

Not everyone who knows how to save knows how to invest the savings wisely, when a certain amount has accumulated. We would like to believe that nurses are not among the dupes, that they are not easily dazzled by so-called gilt-edge investments, that they are wiser than those who embark in the numerous get-rich-quick schemes. But, unfortunately, we have reason to believe that they are not all as wise in the investment of their hard-earned money as they should be.

RULES CONCERNING INVESTMENT

1. Six percent is a liberal return for the use of money.
2. The higher the interest return, the less safe the investment.
3. The personal magnetism of a stock salesman does not add one cent to the value of the stock.
4. Get expert advice concerning investment. You can afford to pay for it, if necessary.
5. Never invest in any new enterprise unless you are willing to devote your own time and energy to it.
6. Never loan a needy friend any more money than you can afford to lose. Your friend probably intends in good faith to pay back the money, but the chances are that he will not be able to repay you.

It is good to have money and the things that money can buy; but it is good, too, to check up once in awhile, and make sure you haven't lost the thing that money can't buy. The spirit of service, the sense of working for a cause that is absolutely worthwhile in which we can spend ourselves without restraint, without reserve, is its own reward. The more of it you give, the richer you become.

To be sure, all nursing is service, but the individual who refuses to render any service for which he is not to receive payment misses much of the joy of living and giving. It should be made a matter of principle every year for a nurse to render a certain amount of service for which she never expects to be paid—and we like to believe that most nurses are carrying out the spirit of this principle and rendering free service in a thousand quiet ways and places.

For Discussion

1. Mention some forms of investment which seem wise for nurses, also the precautions which should be observed.
2. What are the advantages of life insurance as a form of investment for nurses?
3. Suggest some methods by which improvement in present day conditions might be accomplished.

18

THE PIONEER SPIRIT

The pioneer spirit is not dead in the nurses of today, but it is badly in need of better cultivation. The spirit of the pioneer should be in every nurse. She should cultivate the courage to advance beyond the well-populated districts—confident that there is nothing which a brave, healthy, well-trained nurse need fear to meet. There are those who will try to make the pioneer's plans seem ridiculous, who will raise obstacles, and who will hinder by their constant criticism of motives. The real pioneer must be able to go on in spite of difficulties if he expects to accomplish anything worthwhile. The price of pioneering is often unpopularity. Most great causes have at first been unpopular. There will always be those who will urge the life of ease, and urge a nurse not to venture far away.

Stories of heroism and achievement in other lands will lead into new lines of thought and that endeavor will wonderfully enrich the nurse's personal life. From magazines, one can catch glimpses of the manners and customs of people, of their social and sanitary conditions, and their educational methods. The foreign field is calling loudly each year for nurses from America to come take charge of hospitals and dispensaries where health work is so badly needed. They are also teachers of sanitary science, of home economics to the oppressed and down-trodden women, who in many lands are considered simply as chattel property or as slaves. The inspiration, instruction and nursing care that have been so long needed are helping to create in those countries a higher ideal of the value of woman and her place in national life.

No nurse who wishes to be known as well-informed can afford to be ignorant as to the progress in the great movement for the uplift of women that is going on all over the world, a movement in which the nurses of the future are destined to play a more important part.

Every nurse has opportunities to make the world better if she cares to use them. They are everywhere, and great movements often begin with doing some concrete thing that needed to be done at the moment. The established order of things sometimes has to be upset before much progress can be made. There are conditions that are not right in regard to nursing which should be worked at until better conditions are assured. Every epoch-making discovery has implied a way of looking at things differently. The importance of getting a correct viewpoint–to see the needs of the world and what the individual nurse could or should do to meet them, cannot be too strongly emphasized. Civilization advances as new points of view prevail.

Aikens, Charlotte (1916) *Studies in Ethics for Nurses*, Philadelphia: W. B. Saunders Company.

Keep us from pettiness; let us be large in thought, in word, in deed.

Let us be done with fault-finding, and leave off self-seeking.

May we put away all pretense and meet each other face to face—without self-pity and without prejudice.

May we never be hasty in judgment and always generous.

Let us take time for all things; make us to grow calm, serene, gentle.

Teach us to put into action our better impulses, straightforward and unafraid.

Grant that we may realize it is the little things that create differences; that in the big things in life we are at one.

~Mary Stuart